OVERCOMING
RHEUMATISM
AND ARTHRITIS

OVERCOMING RHEUMATISM AND ARTHRITIS

by
PHYLLIS SPEIGHT

Health Science Press
The C.W. Daniel Company Ltd
1 Church Path, Saffron Walden,
Essex, England

By the same author
ARNICA THE WONDER HERB
BEFORE CALLING THE DOCTOR
A COMPARISON OF THE CHRONIC MIASMS
HOMOEOPATHIC REMEDIES FOR CHILDREN
PERTINENT QUESTIONS & ANSWERS
ABOUT HOMOEOPATHY
HOMOEOPATHY FOR EMERGENCIES
A STUDY COURSE IN HOMOEOPATHY
HOMOEOPATHY, A GUIDE TO NATURAL MEDICINE
HOMOEOPATHIC REMEDIES FOR
WOMEN'S AILMENTS
TRANQUILLISATION: THE NON ADDICTIVE WAY
HOMOEOPATHIC REMEDIES FOR
EARS, NOSE AND THROAT
THE TRAVELLER'S GUIDE TO HOMOEOPATHY

This book first published in 1974
Completely revised in 1984
Reprinted 1991

© Phyllis Speight

ISBN 0 85207 166 3

Printed and bound by
Hillman Printers (Frome) Ltd
Frome, Somerset, England

Contents

INTRODUCTION

More and more people suffer from the pains of arthritis and rheumatism.

Special clinics are open to help and prescribe for these unfortunate folk, many of whom become crippled. Yet nothing is heard of any breakthrough in the curing of these ailments. Hopes have been raised with the introduction of drugs such as gold (injections) and cortizone etc., but after a time it is found that comparatively few people derive much benefit, and often side effects develop which can be most unpleasant and, at times, serious.

Let us then turn our attention to a more successful way of combating these chronic and most painful diseases by studying natural remedies and foods.

Much can be done, indeed a great deal has been done, to ease the pains and burdens of the arthritic and rheumatic sufferers but it must be emphasized that the patient should also contribute by adopting some of the suggestions outlined in the following pages.

From experience the writer has found that many patients come for treatment expecting to transfer the responsibility of their illness to the practitioner.

In some ways of course, this is true, but it

does not preclude him from playing his part, a very big part, in co-operating and doing a great deal for himself at home.

Many lessons can and should be learned through illness; it may be patience, or that irritability must be overcome but perhaps the hardest is the lesson of 'acceptance'. This does not mean that the disease is accepted with resignation and a feeling that nothing more can be done; but rather that one should not kick against it, but go along with it and do all in one's power to overcome it.

This cannot be achieved by physical means alone, but by the alteration in thinking to a positive attitude that all will be well.

It must be remembered that no two people are alike, and whilst many complain that they suffer from arthritis or rheumatism, when describing their aches and pains one patient differs a great deal from another. Therefore, many suggestions are given — practical hints that are most important and yet simple to carry out, remedies that may be taken other than drugs, so that no side effects will be experienced, and advice regarding food and drink.

It is the sincere hope of the writer that all who read these pages will put into practice some, if not all of the advice given, and receive benefit.

Chapter 1

RHEUMATISM & ARTHRITIS

There is nothing new about these diseases. In fact examination of Egyptian mummies reveals that rheumatism affected their joints!

No disease is spontaneous. It may seem to appear suddenly in some instances, but in most cases we can trace a chain of symptoms over a long period, many being ignored at the beginning.

But symptoms are not the disease per se — they are only the outward signs of a deeper manifestation in the economy of the patient.

If many of our forebears have suffered from rheumatism or arthritis, then we are born with a blood-stream (soil) which could be suitable for either of these troubles to develop, given the right circumstances.

Sir James Mackenzie put this very aptly many years ago when he gave up a busy practice in Harley Street and retired to a village to study and learn more about preventive medicine.

He came to the conclusion that diseases are the result of long-developing processes, often commencing in childhood and leading to the saturation of toxins in the body.

These same toxins when localized in a joint cause arthritis, when in the liver the disease is called hepatitis; in the kidneys nephritis and so on. This is similar teaching to that of homeopathy.

The homoeopath would add that it is the inherited blood-stream or soil that will channel the toxin to the joints, or to the liver, or to the kidneys.

Poisons begin to build up in the body from an early age due to several factors such as wrong food, unhealthy living habits (lack of exercise, fresh air etc.) and wrong thinking.

The common cold is often nature's way of elimination — remember if children are perfectly healthy they never develop colds!

An attack of influenza, a bad chill, getting soaked through without taking the necessary precautions afterwards, getting overtired and suffering grief or shock are some of the ways in which the body toxins can be wakened into action and then symptoms of a particular disease will appear.

It is, therefore, much wiser to try and cleanse the body by natural means, rather than deal with, and often suppress, the outward signs and symptoms with drugs which can cause side effects and create more problems.

Act Promptly
It cannot be emphasized too strongly that something should be done at the very beginning. So many people say 'Oh I only had a twinge and didn't think any more about it!'

Twinges of pain, stiffness in muscles and joints, backache — all spell out rheumatism in one form or another and the sooner something is done the better.

The daily food should be changed in such a way that acid forming foods are eliminated or cut to the minimum, and only whole foods eaten; they will give maximum minerals,

10

vitamins and substances to build the body and not destroy it. And the question of baths, fresh air and exercise should also be looked into, for not one, but all these factors play a part in helping to bring a 'diseased' body back into a better state of health.

Chapter 2

HOMOEOPATHIC TREATMENT

Dr. John H. Clarke, a world renowned homoeopath, wrote many years ago, 'Homoeopathy, the most complete and scientific system of healing the world has ever seen,' and these facts have been confirmed by homoeopaths all over the world during each succeeding decade.

Today, in spite of modern research, homoeopathy still maintains its supremacy, surviving ridicule by those who had little or no experience of it. There are instances recorded in homoeopathic literature of orthodox doctors setting out to 'debunk' homoeopathy and who, after practical experience, became convinced of its efficacy and adopted it in their practices.

It should be understood that homoeopathy is a system of treatment dealing with the individual patient. Every case is considered separately and the selection of the remedy must be controlled by the symptoms exhibited by the sufferer.

To make this clear let us consider two patients suffering from rheumatism. The first has pain in the lower limbs which are red, swollen, aggravated by heat and worse in the evening. The second has a dull aching in the joints of the wrists and elbows which is aggravated by bathing in cold water. Although both are suffering from rheumatism the symptoms are vastly different and the two patients would be given different remedies in order to overcome their troubles. This is more scientific than 'shot gun' prescribing, consisting of one remedy for every sufferer irrespective of the differing symptoms.

Every homoeopathic remedy has been taken by a number of healthy men and women (called provers) to ascertain the action of each drug on the human economy. After taking a specific remedy for a time, symptoms began to appear and the provers became unwell. Every symptom that was felt or expressed was written down daily. Not only were physical symptoms experienced but those of the mind also, and after a while some provers were on the borderline of insanity. At a given time the proving was stopped and gradually the provers returned to normality, but a very great deal of information had been gathered. These facts were collated and the **Homoeopathic Materia Medica** was built up.

Since the days of Hippocrates it has been known that 'like cures like' but it was Dr. Samuel Hahnemann who developed this knowledge and placed it on a scientific basis with the help of the provers, and the great lesson is that a substance that will cause symptoms in a healthy person will cure similar symptoms in a sick patient.

The same materia medica is still used at the present time for there are no fashions in homoeopathic medicines. Once it is known which symptoms a remedy will cure, this knowledge is for all time, it will never change.

14

In homoeopathic prescribing it is essential to select a remedy that, as near as possible, matches the symptoms of the disease. The more accurate the selection the greater the prospect of success.

When choosing the homoeopathic remedy it is essential to write down the exact location of the ache or pain and a description of it (in the patient's own words); also what makes it better or worse, even though temporarily — e.g. heat, cold, movement, pressure, etc.

Then the remedies should be studied and the one covering the greatest number of symptoms chosen.

An index of symptoms is given near the end of this book for study and help in finding the best remedy to suit the individual set of symptoms.

The name of each homoeopathic remedy followed by a number indicating its strength is recommended in each case. For home prescribing it is advisable to use either the 6th or 12th potency.

The storage of remedies is important. Never leave them in strong sunlight and keep them away from heat and perfumes.

Remedies recommended are those that have achieved great success in the treatment of rheumatic and arthritic ailments but in such a small book it is impossible to include every remedy that might be called for. Should the desired results not be achieved within a reasonable time an experienced homoeopath should be consulted.

One pill of the 6th potency should be taken 3 times daily for 2 weeks, or one pill of the 12th potency night and morning for 2 weeks.

If   1. There is good improvement, then no more medicine should be taken unless the same symptoms return

when it should be repeated.
2. There is slight improvement the remedy should be continued for a further two weeks.
3. Nothing at all has happened the remedy should be changed.

Case Histories

The following case histories will be of interest.

A patient aged 59 years complained of much stiffness and pain across the neck and shoulders. He drove a car every day to and from his office and sat at his desk all day which caused tension in his neck and shoulders. He thought the wet weather had made the condition worse but could not think what had caused it. Apparently it was worse late in the day, and better for movement.

He was given **Rhus t.30** three times a day for three days and three weeks after taking the medicine reported that he was very much better. A little later the same remedy was repeated and nothing was heard of this patient for several months when he asked for more pills as the trouble was returning. Again the prescription was repeated and at the moment all is well.

But it must be pointed out that quite possibly he may need more treatment owing to the fact that until he is 65 and retires, he still has to sit at his office desk doing clerical work, and this does cause muscular tension and stiffness in many people, especially as he has a long drive night and morning.

A woman patient of 64 years of age had been suffering from 'rheumatism' for many months and she had received little relief from drugs.

16

When asked about her aches and pains she found it rather difficult to explain, because, she said, 'I have a bad shooting pain in my arm, then it goes and returns in my leg. Then my foot is sore and the pains seem to move around all the time.'

In answer to some questions she replied that she felt most uncomfortable in great heat but better, and the pains were better, if she could walk about slowly in fresh air.

This case was quite clear cut and the patient was given three doses of **Pulsatilla** in a high potency. Three weeks later she was delighted to be able to say that all her pains had disappeared.

A woman patient of 60 suffered from arthritis in her right wrist. It was very painful and weak so that it was difficult for her to lift anything that was at all heavy. The wrist was swollen and the pain worse on any motion. She was given **Actea spicata 12** night and morning for two weeks and although there was some improvement the trouble did not clear up. She was given the same remedy in a higher potency after which all the swelling and pain disappeared.

About three months later this trouble began to return slightly, but another three doses of this same remedy in a high potency cleared up the trouble and it has not returned.

A patient of 69 years asked for homoeopathic treatment as he was suffering from bad pains in his right knee which made walking difficult. It was very swollen and hot and the pain had begun to go up the leg. The patient said he was worse in the evening and in bed, but he was not sure whether this was due to position or warmth from the bed.

He was given **Ledum 12** night and morning for two weeks and he reported that there was

17

some improvement but the condition was still painful.

Ledum in a higher potency was given and although in another fortnight there was more improvement this condition was not responding as it should have done.

The patient was again questioned closely and this time he remembered that he had strained his knee badly a few weeks previously, but as this seemed to clear up before these pains he did not connect the two.

Calc.c. was given and gradually the swelling disappeared and all the pains abated and have not returned.

Chapter 3

HOMOEOPATHIC REMEDIES

Actea Spicata
This remedy has an affinity with small joints especially of hands and feet. It will help a swollen right wrist when pains are intolerable and slightest pressure on palm causes agony. Excruciating pain in wrist and finger joints, very tender to touch. Severe agonizing pains in joints of fingers, ankles and toes, of a tearing, tingling, drawing character, worse from least motion, or touch, at night.

Small joints swell, are bright red and hot. Swelling of joints after fatigue, patient goes out feeling comfortable but as he walks the joints of his feet ache and swell.

Great stiffness of joints after rest.

Pains as from a paralytic weakness of hands.

The 6th potency should be used.

Ammonium Carbonicum
Should be considered for old people especially women who lead a sedentary life and suffer from gouty rheumatism with great aggravation in winter and wet weather.

Pain in the nape of neck, worse right side; pain under shoulder blades; violent pain in small of back with intense coldness. Right arm heavy, hangs down useless, hand swollen.

Great weakness in lower limbs. Boring and drawing in knees. Cramps in legs; in soles of feet. Heels hurt on standing or walking. Ball of big toe painful and hot. Big toe red, swollen, painful, worse in bed; hot and burning, worse from pressure of shoes. Toes swollen.

All symptoms are better from warmth.

The 6th or 12th potencies should be used.

Antimonium Tartaricum

This is one of the first remedies to be thought of in lumbago when there is violent pain in the the sacro-lumbar region; sometimes it is so severe that the slightest movement causes retching and cold, clammy sweat.

There may be rheumatic pains in the hips, thighs and calves and often the patient is conscious of a bruised sensation in the limbs on and shortly before rising.

Pains in the extremities are sometimes accompanied with sweat which does not relieve.

The sufferer is often in a bad humour; is apprehensive, restless and dreads being alone.

The 12th potency should be used.

Arnica Montana

This is one of the most valuable remedies in articular or muscular rheumatism.

Rheumatism in winter from exposure to dampness and cold; and in strained muscles due to over-exertion. The affected parts feel sore and bruised, worse from any motion, and there is a fear of being touched as it may hurt.

Sharp, shooting pains run down from elbow to forearm or shoot through legs and feet, which often swell and feel sore and bruised.

Limbs ache as if they have been beaten and there may be pain in the intercostal muscles.

Arthritic pains in foot, worse evening. Big toe joint red, feels sprained and very painful; patient is fearful that somebody will kick the painful foot.

A leading symptom of this remedy is that limbs ache as if beaten, and feel sore and bruised.

The 12th potency should be used.

Arsenicum Album

This remedy is often needed in long lasting cases when there is great restlessness of limbs, cannot keep them still, and the pains are burning, shooting and lancinating in character.

Nape of neck feels stiff as if bruised or sprained.

Neuralgic pains on left side of neck

Tearing, jerking pains in right shoulder joint and shoulder.

Pains in the arm on the side one lies on at night.

Drawing, jerking and tearing from the tips of the fingers into the shoulders.

Backache after hard work. Burning in back.

Stiffness and immobility of knees and feet. Coldness of knees and feet.

There is often great debility of the patient, sometimes with faintness; there is also restlessness and anxiety especially at night.

The 12th potency should be used.

Bryonia Alba

This remedy should be thought of in all types of rheumatic troubles when:

1. They are worse from any motion.
2. There is relief from lying on the painful side.
3. There is a marked improvement from perspiring.

In muscular rheumatism the muscles are sore to touch and sometimes swollen, worse from slightest motion. Both joints and fibrous tissues may be involved.

Arthritic joints are hot, red, swollen, stinging and stiff with stitching pains.

Bryonia should be thought of when there are stitching, stabbing pains in intercostal muscles.

Tearing pains in right shoulder joint and arms with tension and stitches and shining red swellings.

Stitches in knee when walking.

Stitches in knee joint with pain in ligaments.

Feet tense and swollen in evening.

Gouty swelling of heel with redness, heat and much pain.

Always consider this remedy when there is rheumatism with redness and swelling of joints and the least movement causes severe pain; pains are worse morning and evening.

There is an amelioration while sitting, lying on painful side, from warmth of bed and from sweating.

The 6th potency should be used.

Calcarea Carbonica

This is of great value in chronic rheumatism of the joints. It helps rheumatism from working in water; and chronic cases with swelling of joints worse with every change of weather.

Rheumatic pains in the limbs associated with much stiffness.

The neck becomes stiff and rigid after over-straining or lifting.

Pain in the whole of back as if strained. Stitches or pressive pains in dorsal region of back.

Arthritic pain in right wrist as if it had been dislocated.

Hands and forearms feel cramped in morning, swelling of hands.

Arthritic nodes on hands and fingers.

Sciatic pains from working in cold water.

Stitching and tearing in knees. Knee swollen, red, hot, with pain through whole limb on motion. Great swelling of the knee joint. Spongy swelling of knee joint.

Pain in calf on walking; knotty cramps in calves.

There is often a sensation as if cold wet stockings were on the feet.

All pains are worse in cold, wet weather, in the morning, when ascending, after eating, from walking and working in water.

The 12th potency should be used.

Caulophyllum Thalictroides
This is one of the most valuable remedies in rheumatic conditions affecting the small joints, especially wrists, ankles, fingers and toes. It is almost always associated with a deranged female sexual system.

This should be compared with **Actea Spicata.**

It should be thought of in rheumatism of wrists and fingers joints with swelling and cutting pains in joints when closing the hands.

Pains often shift to nape of neck, with rigidity and oppression of chest; in fact pains do not remain long in any one place before moving to another.

The 6th potency should be used.

Causticum

Arthritic pains in all limbs. Chronic articular rheumatism when joints are stiff and tendons shortened, drawing the limbs out of shape, worse from cold and better by warmth; restless at night; averse to being uncovered.

Stiffness of neck, cannot move head.

Painful stiffness of back especially on rising from chair.

Rheumatic aching in shoulder. Dull drawing and tearing in forearms and hands. Contractions and indurations of tendons of fingers. Nodes. Toes or fingers contracted.

Stitching pains in hip joints. Drawing and tearing in thighs and legs, knees and feet worse in open air, better in warmth of bed. Cracking in knees when walking. Tension in knees and ankle joints. Crawling, burning and severe pressive pains in ball of big toe.

Paralytic weakness of limbs.

Continual tearing and piercing pains compelling constant motion which does not relieve; always coming on in the evening and diminishing in the morning.

Cold dry winds and draughts aggravate symptoms but warm, moist weather gives relief.

The 6th potency should be used.

Cimicifuga (Actea Racemosa)

This is a valuable remedy in muscular rheumatism affecting the belly of the muscles, especially those of the neck, back and chest.

Rheumatic pains in muscles of neck and back with feeling of stiffness and contraction. Rheumatism of dorsal muscle. Severe pains in small of back extending down thighs. Violent aching in lumbar region.

Severe pains down arms with numbness as if a nerve had been compressed.

Joints feel stiff, especially at night and in the morning.

Pains are worse on motion and better from rest.

The 6th potency should be used.

Colchicum

This remedy has a special affinity with fibrous tissues, tendons and ligaments of joints and periosteum, but its action is more marked in relation to the small joints. Rheumatism and arthritis of the small joints of the hands and feet, especially of the big toes, where the pains are sharp and sticking are often helped by this remedy.

These pains often move from joint to joint and are worse from both heat and cold, especially damp cold. They are worse from least touch or jar which induces a fear of being approached. Remember **Colchicum** for rheumatic pains in the shoulders, arms and back of neck preventing motion of head.

There are often tearing pains in muscles and joints; and stiff neck with paroxysms of anguish.

The 12th potency should be used.

Colocynthis

Think of this remedy in rheumatism with tearing or drawing pains in all limbs which motion generally relieves.

There is stiffness of the joints; stiffness in the muscles of the nape of the neck when moving the head.

Drawing, lancinating pains attack the left shoulder from face to neck. Rheumatic pains occur in arms, and tearing in joint of left hand. There is pain in thumb impeding motion, and violent, drawing pain in right thumb.

Cramping pains sometimes occur in affected hip as though the part were screwed in a vice; pain as if hips were screwed together. Pain in right thigh only when walking. Continuous pain in left knee joint impeding walking.

Drawing, aching in left foot.

The pains are worse by movement and eased by warmth.

The 12th potency should be used.

Eupatorium Perfoliatum

Is very useful in rheumatic troubles accompanied by perspiration and great soreness of the muscles and bones.

Pain in neck and back of head. Weakness and intolerable aching soreness as if beaten in small of back. Bruised or intense pain in back.

Sensation as if arm had been beaten above and below elbow. Pain in both wrists as if broken or dislocated.

Rheumatic pain on inside of left knee; soreness and aching in lower limbs; stiffness and general soreness on rising to walk. Calves feel as if they have been beaten. Pain in first joint of left big toe then it suddenly shifts to the other foot. Intolerable pain under toe nails.

Gouty inflammation of left knee and right elbow.

All symptoms are worse in the morning and on motion.

The 6th potency should be used.

Gelsemium
This is a remedy which gives good service in muscular rheumatism.

Pains in the neck can be severe, and under the left shoulder blade. Bruised pains in muscles of neck.

There is often dull aching in lumbar and sacral regions.

Deep seated dull aching pain in limbs and joints is often brought on by cold.

This remedy should be thought of when there is great fatigue of limbs after slight exertion.

Complaints follow bad or exciting news. There is complete relaxation of whole muscular system. Patient feels very tired, even the eyelids feel heavy and tired.

The 12th potency should be used.

Gnaphalium Polycephalum
This is a marvellous remedy when there is intense pain along the sciatic nerve alternating with numbness.

It is also recommended for chronic backache in lumbar region with numbness.

The 6th or 12th potencies should be used.

Hepar Sulphuris
This remedy should be thought of when rheumatic troubles result from exposure to cold, dry winds, or when the joints are affected.

Drawing pains between the shoulder blades. Bruised sensation in small of back and lumbar region. Pain in shoulder as if a weight were resting on it.

Tearing in arms. Hot, red swelling of joints

27

of fingers and hands, with stiffness.

Sensation of soreness in thighs. Bruised pain and swelling of knee joint; swelling of ankle. Cramps in soles and toes.

Worse at night; cold, dry air; cold winds.

Better from warmth and wrapping up warmly.

The 6th potency should be used.

Ledum Palustre

It is easy to match this remedy to the symptoms it will cure because its characteristics are so pronounced.

The rheumatic pains go from below upward; the joints are pale, swollen and tense; the pains are hot, stinging and drawing, worse warmth of bedclothes, motion and evening.

Gouty rheumatism begins in lower limbs and ascends. Joints have large amounts of nodes in them.

There are rending pains in periosteum, swelling of feet and legs up to knees. Skin is purple and mottled. These symptoms are better when holding feet in ice water.

Gout with tearing pains in toes; gouty nodosities in joints.

Pain in ankles as from a severe strain or mis-step.

Ball of big toe painful, swollen, tendons stiff worse stepping.

The 12th potency should be used.

Magnesium Carbonica

Is especially suitable for children who are very irritable, nervous and sour smelling; and for 'worn out women' who are spare, thin and sensitive.

Much pain in right shoulder, can scarcely raise arm; pain as if dislocated in shoulder joint. Pain in shoulder with tingling down fingers which prevents least motion, worse at night. Red swelling of fingers.

Drawing pain in legs and feet. Pains around left knee with tightness.

Can stand but cannot walk. Swelling in bend of knee very painful. Knees painful when walking, feet when lying in bed.

Worse draughts, change of temperature.

Better warmth.

The 6th potency should be used.

Natrum Muriaticum

Has marked rigidity of all joints. Painful stiffness of neck. Spine oversensitive to touch or pressure. Pain in back from stooping, worse while straightening up. Bruised pain. Shoulder joint feels sprained. Stitches in muscles and joints of hands and fingers. Moves finger joints with difficulty.

Pain in hip as if sprained. Stitches in right hip joint. Drawing pain in right thigh extending to knee. Painful tension in bend of limbs.

Sprained pain in knee and ankles. Housemaids' knee. Lameness in ankle joint. Big toe red with tearing and stinging. Stiffness and arthritic swellings. Worse sitting, walking and at night. Better lying on something hard. This patient is often very fond of salt.

The 6th or 12th potencies should be used.

Nux Vomica

The call for this remedy may be for almost any form of rheumatism, when associated with the great leading symptoms; worse from cold, from 3 to 4 a.m., patient is over sensitive to all reactions, has marked nervous debility and excitement, is very irritable and constipated, with ineffectual urging. Nux patients like rain and cloudy weather. They feel better on a warm, muggy grey day.

If any of these marked symptoms are present **Nux Vomica** will help stiff neck with heaviness, backache when patients has to sit up to turn over in bed; bruised pains in small of back or lumbago which comes on from cold with acute spasmodic pain, and bruised heavy pains in shoulders.

The pains are aching, drawing and bruised. Worse any motion; cold.

Better warmth and hot drinks.

Rheumatism or arthritis usually attacks the muscles of the trunk and large joints. The swellings are pale with numbness and twitching.

The 12th potency should be used.

Phytolacca
This remedy should be considered for the following:- Stiff neck on the right side; back very stiff every morning in damp weather; pains extending up and down back; pains go up the neck to back of head. Pains in small of back in lumbar muscles. Constant dull, heavy pains in lumbar and sacral region. Lumbago. Back is very stiff every morning. Rheumatic pains shoot from sacrum down both legs.

Aching in both shoulders and arms; pains fly like electric shocks from one part to another.

Rheumatic, drawing pains in both arms; inability to raise arm.

Chronic rheumatism in left hip joint, and lower limbs.

Rheumatic pain in right knee, worse open air and damp weather.

Chronic gouty inflammation of both knee

joints. Pains in bones of legs at night.
Gouty pains in big toe.

All pains are worse motion, damp weather, at night and sitting.

The 6th potency should be used.

Pulsatilla

The pains of rheumatism which are helped by this remedy are often caused by getting wet, especially the feet, and by protracted hot weather.

They are wandering pains and shift rapidly from one part to another. Symptoms are constantly changing.

There may be drawing, tensive pain in nape of neck. Back painful and stiff; pain in small of back on motion as if sprained. Constricted pain in small of back. Lumbago compelling patient to move, yet motion brings no relief.

Drawing, tearing, jerking pains may develop in shoulder joints and arms; are painful when at rest extending down to thumb. Swelling sometimes occurs in joints of hand with redness.

The hip joint can be very painful and feel as if dislocated and there may be drawing and tension in thighs and legs.

Pains in knee are tearing, jerking, drawing and shooting with swelling and inflammation. Feet red, inflamed and swollen; boring pains in heels.

All aches and pains are worse at night, from warmth and are better for uncovering. Patient often gets out of bed in the night to cool down.

Patients needing this remedy are often indecisive, easily moved to tears, and have a great desire for open air.

The 6th potency should be used.

Ranunculus Bulbosus

This remedy has helped many cases of muscular rheumatism of the chest, and intercostal rheumatism where there is marked soreness to touch, as if the muscles had been pounded.

The pains are stitching and of a neuralgic type. Stitches about chest with every change of weather; rheumatism of chest and abdominal muscles due to exposure; with a bruised pain increasing to sharp cutting pain.

Ranunculus should also be remembered when there is pain along the inner edge of left scapula.

There may be burning sensation and pain in the back as if bruised often accompanied by burning.

There may be rheumatic and arthritic soreness with stitches all over the body.

All pains are worse lying down, in the evening, on entering a cold room, change of weather, wet days and during storms.

The 6th potency should be used.

Rhododendron

This remedy is useful in early summer when the weather is cold and damp for the time of year, with cold winds and storms.

Pains in back and shoulders, stiff neck, pains fly in all directions.

Violent, tearing, boring pains in left shoulder joint with prickling of fingers. Tearing, cramp-like, drawing in forearm. Sensation as if wrists were strained.

Periodical tearing in lower limbs especially about hip joint.

Affection of big toe joint of a rheumatic character often mistaken for a bunion.

Arthritic nodes.

Chronic rheumatism affecting the small joints and their ligaments.

Worse motion; thunderstorms; vexation; cold weather; wind.

The 6th or 12th potencies should be used.

Rhus Toxicodendron

This is one of the most valuable remedies in every form of rheumatism. It acts on the fibrous tissue and sheaths of muscles.

Chief symptoms in the rheumatic field are stiff neck with painful tension. Pain in shoulders and back with stiffness as from a sprain. Stiffness or aching, or bruised pain in small of back whilst sitting or lying. Heaviness and pressure in small of back as if patient had received a heavy blow. Violent pain in lumbar region as if back were broken.

Violent tearing pain in arm, worse lying still. Aching and numbness in left arm. Chronic articular inflammation resulting from sprains.

Jerking, tearing in elbow and wrist joints. Rheumatic pains and swelling of hands, especially during wet weather. Motion of fingers painful, can only move them with pain because of swelling.

Pressive pains in hip joint; tearing and drawing from hip to knee while walking or standing.

Dull, aching pain in right sciatic nerve, stiffness of knees and feet. Aching pains in feet, unable to rest.

There is a sense of stiffness on first moving the part after rest. Pains are drawing or tearing during rest; bruised or sprained in the joints. Joints crack when moved. Rheumatoid pains in limbs with numbness and tingling. Joints are weak; stiff or red, shining and swollen.

All pains are worse from draughts; when beginning to move; sitting; lying quietly; lying

33

on something hard; after motion, cold, wet weather; damp weather and at night.

They are better by rubbing, heat and when warmed by exercise. They love warm applications, leaning against a warm pad.

The patient needing this remedy is often very restless, constantly wanting to move the affected part; has great debility with soreness and stiffness; twitching of limbs; and a rheumatic diathesis.

The 12th potency should be used.

Ruta Graveolens

This remedy is capable of clearing up many rheumatic pains which follow injury to bones. The patient always complains of bruised and sprained pains.

Rheumatic pains in back. Bruised pain in lumbar region. Pain as from a fall or blow in back and coccyx.

Lameness after sprains especially of wrists and ankles.

Hip bones feel bruised.

All pains are worse cold damp weather; sitting or lying; cold applications.

The 6th potency should be used.

Sanguinaria Canadensis

This remedy has an affinity with the right arm and shoulder and has cleared up many rheumatic and arthritic pains in this area, which are worse at night, worse on turning in bed and when the patient cannot raise his arm. There is also pain in top of right shoulder.

There are also rheumatic pains in nape of neck, shoulders and arms, lumbago from lifting and pain in large muscles of back. These rheumatic pains are worse in places least covered with flesh. Rheumatism in all joints with swelling and spasmodic pain; rheuma-

34

tism in all limbs with stiffness and rigidity.

It is also excellent in acute inflammatory and arthritic rheumatism.

All pains are worse from lifting, at night, when turning in bed, on motion and in hot weather.

The 6th potency should be used.

Sulphur

This remedy is indicated when the patient cannot walk erect; he stoops or bends forward when walking or sitting. There is often acute pain in small of back making rising from a seat difficult; this has to be done slowly. There is a sensation that everything is too short. Rheumatic pains in shoulders — the left is worst and there is a great desire to keep the arm moving for relief. Hands are hot and sweaty. Pains are worse at night. There may be arthritic swellings in knee joints which crack on motion. The ankle joints are very stiff.

Rheumatic conditions are continually relapsing. There may be an offensive odour of the body.

Intense burning occurs in affected parts, the feet often burn in bed and patient wants to find a cool place for them. He is very sensitive to open air. Will not bath more often than he has to.

The patient needing this remedy does not enjoy hot weather.

The 6th potency should be used.

TO ASSIST IN THE SELECTION OF THE CORRECT HOMOEOPATHIC REMEDY THERE IS A HOMOEOPATHIC INDEX OF SYMPTOMS ON PAGE 80.

Chapter 4

CORRECT DIET IS ESSENTIAL

Contrary to general opinion a correct diet is of greater importance than most people think.

More and more people realize the importance of eating 'whole' foods but, unfortunately, there are still some who consume quantities of packeted, tinned, fried and junk foods washed down with copious cups of strong tea and coffee, sweetened with spoonsful of white sugar.

Most of us make many errors, as far as food is concerned. We may eat a great deal too much, or eat things we most enjoy, regardless of whether there is any real value in them for building and maintaining the body.

Much of our food is de-vitalized; it is grown in artificial fertilizers; processed, coloured and often tinned. Roughage, so good for the bowel, is removed and mineral salts boiled out in cooking or swamped by the addition of too much salt or sugar.

All white flour products should be eliminated. This is because the wheat germ, minerals and substances vital to health have been refined out during the milling processes, which means that the product is much less wholesome.

Therefore all bread, pastries, cakes, buns,

scones and biscuits made from white flour should be avoided.

Instead 100 per cent wholemeal bread should be eaten; this is delicious, has a nutty flavour and is much more satisfying. Wholemeal flour contains the wheatgerm which is a good source of vitamin B1 and E and is rich in iron and phosphorus. Roughage also is contained in this flour which is so good for the bowel.

Sugar should be cut to a minimum and white sugar never used, because through the refining stages all the vital minerals and trace elements are removed, leaving a sweetening agent which is very acid. It is very important for arthritic and rheumatic patients to take heed of this advice; many physicians of the orthodox school are in agreement here.

Honey is the best natural sweetener but even this should be used sparingly.

Salads

The more raw food that is eaten the better, and a large salad should be taken every day. This is cleansing and contains many natural vitamins and mineral salts and, with a little protein such as grated nuts, grated cheese, cream or cottage cheese, or olives and perhaps the addition of slices of orange, apple, pear or banana, a delicious meal is created. The salad should comprise lettuce or watercress, with perhaps four, five or six other ingredients as follows, grated raw carrot or beetroot, radishes, tomatoes, cucumber unpeeled, celery, onions, grated heart of cabbage, or grated brussels sprouts. Herbs such as chopped chives, parsley and mint all add flavour. Sunflower seeds are good in any salad.

A french dressing can be made by blending the juice of one lemon with 4-5 tablespoonsful of sunflower oil, salt and pepper to taste.

Put all ingredients in a screw top jar and shake well. Store in refrigerator.

OR, half-a-pint of natural yoghourt combined with juice and rind of half a lemon, half a teaspoon of honey, one tablespoon of finely chopped onion, salt and pepper to taste. Mix as above.

Avocado pears are delicious in any salad and they contain, as do nuts, an oil similar to the synovial fluid natural to the joints of the body.

Vegetables should be conservatively cooked either by steaming or in a Pyrex dish with a tightly fitting lid, in the oven. They must never be boiled in lots of water, soda should never be added and only the minimum amount of salt.

Never cook in aluminium saucepans — see supplementary advice.

Fruit except rhubarb and gooseberries should be eaten raw when possible. If cooked, a little honey may be added for sweetening.

Unless vegetarian, a little roast lamb, chicken or white fish may be taken with potatoes baked in their jackets or steamed unpeeled (the latter may be skinned when cooked if desired as then the paper-like outer covering will come away easily without disturbing the mineral salts etc., which are just underneath). A green vegetable and some carrots will complete the course. A cooked vegetarian dish may replace meat and fish.

Care should be taken not to mix the wrong foods at any one meal. For instance protein (meat, poultry, fish, eggs, cheese and nuts) should be eaten with conservatively cooked green vegetables and a jacket potato and followed by fruit, raw or cooked. (If a vegetarian savoury of a starchy nature is the protein dish then the jacket potato should be omitted.)

Starches and proteins should not be taken at the same meal.

Tea, coffee, cocoa and alcohol should be eliminated from the diet, and this is important for the first three months anyway; after that a cup of weak China tea may be taken occasionally and a cup of coffee very infrequently. Alcohol should be taken very sparingly. Instead, herbal teas are excellent, see Chapter 7. Fruit juices are cleansing, and if hot drinks are desired in cold weather yeast extract can be used.

Milk is a clogging, mucus-forming food and should not be consumed in any quantity. Milky drinks are not good taken at bedtime. Hot lemon sweetened with a little honey, or one of the herbal teas should be substituted.

Foods containing potassium should be taken where possible as most people suffering from arthritis and rheumatism are lacking in this mineral. They include celery, avocado pears, apples, bananas, cherries, dates, dried figs and peaches, potatoes in their jackets, whole wheat, almonds, cottage cheese, watercress, lentils, raisins and grapes.

Potassium Broth

The following recipe for Potassium Broth is cleansing and contains many mineral salts as well as potassium; it is also alkaline.

Clean and prepare 2 cupsful of finely chopped or grated:-

> Carrot or turnip
> Spinach or watercress
> Onion or leeks
> Tomato, fresh or bottled
> Celery or 1 tablespoon crushed celery seeds
> Parsley — ¼ of a cupful only

Place in an enamel or stainless steel saucepan with 5 pints of water, bring to the boil and simmer for at least 20 minutes. Then add 2 teaspoonsful of yeast extract for flavouring. This delicious drink may be taken mid-morning or before the evening meal.

Salt should be avoided. Many people eat far too much salt and any excess of bodily needs puts great strain on the kidneys as it has to be eliminated. There is sufficient salt in ordinary foods for the requirements of the body and therefore it is unwise to add more.

To be avoided are — all spices and highly-seasoned food; jam, pickles, sausages, canned meats, canned fruits (because of the thick sugar syrup), all fried foods, sweets, chocolates and ice-creams; all manufactured packeted foods, artificial colourings and flavours.

Detoxifying Daily Diet
The following is a typical daily diet which should be taken to help the body rid itself of toxins.

On waking	A glass of diluted fruit juice, or lemon and raisin drink if constipated (see Chapter 9).
Breakfast	2 raw apples or pears, or a dish comprising grated raw apple or pear with 2 dessertspoonsful of bran and one of a wheat germ product; a teaspoonful (or 2 if desired) of honey or crude black molasses with diluted fruit juice, or the breakfast dish given in Chapter 9.
Mid-morning	A cup of potassium broth, dandelion coffee or herb tea.

Midday meal	A good mixed salad (details given earlier in this chapter) with a wholemeal biscuit or slice of wholemeal bread with butter or vegetarian margarine. This may be followed by fresh fruit or some dates, raisins, sultanas or a junket or yoghourt.
Tea-time	Cup of herb tea.
Evening meal	A cup of potassium broth or some vegetable soup followed by a savoury vegetarian dish, with two or three steamed green vegetables, carrots and jacket potatoes. If non-vegetarian a little lamb, chicken or fish (not fried) may be eaten. For a sweet follow the midday meal, or baked apples may be sweetened with a little honey. The centres of baked apples may be filled with raisins, sultanas, and nuts etc. Occasionally an egg custard or some natural yoghourt may be taken.
Bedtime drink	A cup of herb tea, hot yeast extract drink or weak dandelion coffee with very little milk.

The midday and evening meal may be changed if convenient. Another diet that is somewhat different but interesting is that of Dr. Dong. He prohibits the intake of dairy foods and meat but encourages his patients to eat plenty of fish and a little chicken. He recommends all vegetables except tomatoes. Full details are given in two books on his regime entitled NEW HOPE FOR THE ARTHRITIC by Dr. Colin H. Dong and Jane Banks and THE ARTHRITIC'S COOKBOOK by the same authors. Many people have derived great benefit from his diet.

Chapter 5

VITAMINS

Vitamins are essential for good health and should be taken by everybody, preferably in our daily food. Unhappily, however, this is not possible as very few people are able to obtain sufficient natural foods because so many are processed and refined to such an extent that hardly any vitamins or trace elements are left.

Quite often it is necessary to prescribe a course of vitamins but it is a mistake to believe that the taking of one or more will cure most diseases; neither must they be taken indefinitely, for too many are almost as bad as a deficiency.

It should be understood that natural vitamins are referred to here and not the synthetic varieties.

Vitamin C

This vitamin is important as it helps to keep the body healthy. Experiments have shown that when a person is sick no vitamin C is found in the blood or urine, but the more vitamin C the sick patient consumes, generally, more progress is made. It appears that the toxic substances combine with this vitamin and the two are excreted together in the urine. Obviously a great deal more vitamin C is needed when a person is sick than when healthy.

This is one of the reasons why vitamin C is so necessary for arthritic and rheumatic patients. Another is that it helps to form Calcium citrate with food containing Calcium and so makes it possible (together with other body activities) for the body to use the Calcium in building firm bones, teeth, cartilage and healthy capillaries.

The richest sources of vitamin C are found in rose-hips, turnip-tops, sprouts, dandelion leaves, grapefruit, oranges, cabbage, blackcurrants, strawberries, kale, broccoli, parsley, watercress and tomatoes.

Natural vitamin C tablets are available containing 500 or 1000mgs (and less of course) and I would recommend 1000mgs to be taken in the morning and 1000mgs at bedtime because this vitamin remains in the body for only 10 to 11 hours.

If you take too many aspirins much vitamin C is lost from the body.

Vitamin B Complex

The B vitamins help the nervous system but they need to be taken together for maximum results and, therefore, the B complex is recommended. One tablet 3 times daily of 100mgs for a period followed by a short rest.

Vitamin E

Most people benefit from vitamin E as it helps to alleviate fatigue, acts as a diuretic, supplies oxygen to the body and retards cellular ageing.

Best natural sources. Wheat germ, soya beans, vegetable oils, broccoli, brussels sprouts, leafy greens, spinach, wholewheat, whole grain cereals and eggs.

400ius of vitamin E daily is an average dose but those with high blood pressure or a history of rheumatic fever should begin with very small doses, e.g. 100ius and increase by 100 every 10 to 14 days.

Vitamin E strengthens the heart before dilating the capillaries.

Cooking in copper pots can destroy vitamin E. Chlorinated water destroys this vitamin.

Calcium and Phosphorus

Calcium and Phosphorus tablets (2 parts calcium and 1 of phosphorus) have been found to reduce pain in some cases of arthritis and rheumatism.

Calcium also helps the body to use iron.

Vitamin D is necessary to enable the body to obtain the full benefit of calcium and some tablets include this.

Natural sources of calcium are milk and dairy products, cheese, peanuts, sunflower seeds, walnuts, soybeans, dried beans, green vegetables, salmon and sardines.

With most calcium supplements a small dose of vitamin A is helpful but not large doses; the body can store vitamin A so a daily intake in unnecessary.

Natural sources of vitamin A are green and yellow vegetables, yellow fruits, fish liver oil, eggs, milk and cheese.

Devil's Claw (Harpagophytum procumbens)

There are many reports in this country showing that improvement has taken place in cases of arthritis after the patients have taken Devil's Claw tablets.

If the urine tends to become dark brown while taking this treatment there is no need for anxiety, it is, in fact, the body eliminating toxic matter.

Follow the dosage on the package.

Garlic

Garlic is recommended because it helps to cleanse the blood of impurities and this can only be helpful.

It is advisable to wash down the capsules with a cold drink otherwise it can repeat.

Again follow directions of dosage on packet.

Selenium

Selenium is a very rare trace element found in varying degrees in the soil but vast areas in the world including Great Britain have very little concentration and so anything grown in these areas will be lacking in this element which is important for our health.

Experiments have shown that a number of chronic sufferers from arthritis and rheumatism whose aches and pains have not been alleviated by drugs, have vastly improved after taking selenium.

It works better with vitamin E and like that vitamin it's an anti-oxidant.

Natural sources are bran, wheatgerm, tuna fish, tomatoes, onions and broccoli.

Dosage is recommended on package.

It is again emphasised, however, that vitamins are an excellent supplement, they play their part and are a facet of natural healing.

Chapter 6

HERBAL MEDICINE

This is the oldest form of medicine known to man.

Hippocrates, who is recognised as the 'Father of Medicine' lived in the fourth century B.C. and in his writings are records of herbs in the treatment of disease.

They played a very great part in treating the sick during the Middle Ages and quotations from old herbals help us to understand the amazing work done by herbalists in far off days.

There seems to be a reviving interest in herbal medicine once again due, no doubt, to the fact that so many people find that drugging is not the answer.

Herbs are natural remedies containing not only healing properties, but minerals and vitamins which have a profound influence on the human economy — the blood, nerves, glands, metabolism and all the processes vital to life.

Their action is safe and soothing, they do not suppress and have no side effects.

Most herbs have more than one action. For instance chamomile expels flatulence, calms the nervous system and acts as a tonic. Cinnamon is aromatic, it causes contractions of the tissues, produces energy and eases griping

47

pains and flatulence. Irish moss soothes the whole of the alimentary tract, helps the chest and lungs and is nourishing.

Herbs are foods as well as medicines because they contain starches, sugars and protein.

They may be taken over a long period and in conjunction with homoeopathic remedies.

The following list of herbs is a very brief one, owing to limited space, but it is certain that regular doses of herbal remedies over a long period will help to remove excess uric acid from the system, aid digestion and bowel movement, tone up the system generally and supply more energy.

Herbal teas should be substituted where possible for ordinary tea and coffee. They are pleasant and refreshing and help to purify the blood. They can be made in a teapot just as ordinary tea which is quick and simple.

The following should be studied carefully and the most appropriate herb or herbs taken daily.

Birch (Betula alba)
Bitter, astringent.

Coleridge talks of this tree as the 'Lady of the Woods'; it is very elegant and after rain gives off a fragrant odour.

The young shoots, leaves and bark are all used for healing purposes but the leaves help to ease the pains of rheumatism and gout.

A pint of boiling water should be added to 1oz of the dried leaves and left to cool. When strained a wineglassful should be taken 3 times daily.

Burdock (Arctium lappa)
Diaphoretic, diuretic.

The flowers of this herb are like thistles,

purple in colour, globular, with burrs that can stick to clothing!

The herb, roots and seeds (which are really the fruits) all contain healing properties. It is one of the finest blood purifiers in herbal medicine. It is very rich in iron.

It is said that burdock seeds carried in a muslin bag around the neck help to keep rheumatism at bay. Be that as it may, a decoction from the root is helpful in all rheumatic troubles.

A decoction of both the root and seeds should be prepared in the proportion of 1oz to 1½ pints of water boiled down to 1 pint. A wineglassful should be taken 3 or 4 times daily.

Celery (Apium graveolens)

Carminative, diuretic and tonic.

This is a most important remedy for rheumatic troubles and its virtues have been known for many years. In 1879 The Times published a letter written by Mr. Gibson Ward who was at that time President of The Vegetarian Society in which he said, 'Celery, when cooked is a very fine dish, both as nutriment and as a purifier of the blood. . . . Let me fearlessly say that rheumatism is impossible on this diet.'

Celery juice is probably a solvent of uric acid which makes it such an important remedy for rheumatic disorders.

The sticks should be washed and stewed well in not too much water, strained and a wineglassful taken 3 times daily.

If fresh celery is unobtainable (it is usually available at greengrocers nearly all the year now it is imported from abroad) celery seeds may be used. They should be stewed gently for about three hours. The liquid should be

49

strained and a wineglassful taken 3 times daily.

Centaury (Erythraea centaurium)
Aromatic, bitter, stomachic, tonic.

This herb purifies the blood and also acts as a tonic. It formed the basis of the once famous Portland Powder which was said to be a specific for gout. It is most helpful in dealing with muscular rheumatism.

An infusion is made by pouring one pint of boiling water onto 1oz of the dried herb and when cold and strained a wineglassful should be taken 2 or 3 times daily.

Dandelion (Taraxicum officinale)
Diuretic, tonic and slightly aperient.

The bright yellow flowers are familiar to us all. When picked and used when fresh they make a delicious wine.

This herb is an excellent blood purifier and the young leaves should be added to salads. The older leaves are very bitter and must be avoided.

Dandelion coffee made from the ground roasted roots is very good and beneficial to health. It is slightly laxative.

This herb is rich in mineral salts and among others it contains calcium, iron, magnesium, potassium, silicon and sodium and has been used to help arthritic sufferers as it promotes the removal of uric acid from the blood.

1oz of the root should be boiled in 1½ pints of water for 30 minutes. This should then be strained and a wineglassful taken night and morning.

Goutwort (Aegopodium podagraria)
Diuretic, sedative.

This herb grows like a weed and is found

near monasteries having been introduced by the monks.

Culpeper states, 'It is probable that the name of Gout Herb from its peculiar virtues in healing the cold gout and sciatica as it hath been found by experience to be a most admirable remedy for these disorders. . . . It is even affirmed that the very carrying of it about in the pocket will defend the bearer from any attack of the aforesaid complaint.'

The herb is a sedative and used to allay painful joints in rheumatism and gout.

The young leaves are eaten as a green vegetable in Switzerland; they make a good hot compress for rheumatic pains — follow the directions given under Horseradish.

The liquid extract should be obtained and ½ to 1 teaspoonful taken in water twice daily.

Guaiacum (Guaiacum officinale)
Diaphoretic, alterative.

Another name for Guaiacum is 'Lignum Vitae' which is an ornamental evergreen tree which grows in the West Indian Islands and north coast of South America.

The wood from this tree is very hard and heavy and the 'woods' used in bowls are made from it, as are skittle boards, some rulers etc.

The resin from the wood has medical properties and is especially useful in rheumatoid arthritis, chronic rheumatism and gout.

It has a reputation of relieving the pain and inflammation; and helps to remove impurities from the blood.

The liquid extract may be obtained from most health food stores and ½ to 1 teaspoonful in water should be taken twice daily.

Hops (Humulus lupulus)
Tonic, anodyne, diuretic, aromatic, bitter.

As an external remedy a fomentation made from hops and chamomile flowers removes the pain and allays inflammation, and neuralgic and muscular pains in muscular rheumatism.

The fomentation should be made by pouring sufficient boiling water onto a handful of hops and chamomile flowers to make them moist and hot, then the remaining water should be squeezed out, and the flowers placed between two layers of linen and applied to the affected part. This may be repeated as often as is necessary. Care should be taken not to burn the skin.

Horseradish (Cochlearia armoracia)
Stimulant, diaphoretic, diuretic.

This herb contains a large proportion of sulphur and is recommended used externally in chronic rheumatism.

Culpeper says, 'If bruised and laid to a part grieved with Sciatica, gout, joint-ache or hard swellings of the spleen and liver, it doth wonderfully help them all.'

A compress is made by grating the root and covering with sufficient hot milk to make into a paste. Put this between two layers of linen and apply to the affected part while still warm.

It is best to apply the poultice at night in order that it may be left in place all night.

Juniper Berries (Juniperus communia)
Diuretic, stimulant, carminative.

This herb is usually prescribed for diseases of the kidney and bladder but it has the power to increase the excretion of uric acid through the urine and so is helpful in all forms of arthritis and rheumatism.

Dr. Fernie explained that '. . . . if applied externally to painful local swellings whether rheumatic or neuralgic the bruised berries will afford prompt and lasting relief.'

The infusion, which stimulates most bodily functions is made by adding one pint of boiling water to 1oz of berries and when strained wineglass doses taken three times daily.

Nettle (Urtica dioica)
Diuretic, astringent, tonic.

This weed has many properties beneficial to the body and the very young nettle tops should be gathered, cooked and eaten like spinach.

The nettle is an excellent blood purifier and a solvent of uric acid and therefore especially good for patients suffering from rheumatism and arthritis.

One pint of boiling water should be poured onto 1oz of the fresh or dried herb, strained when cold and a wineglassful taken three times daily.

Prickly Ash (Xanthoxylum americanum)
Stimulant, alterative, tonic, diaphoretic.

Berries - also carminative and antispasmodic.

The bark and berries are both valuable as medicine, removing impurities from the blood.

Prickly Ash is greatly recommended in chronic rheumatism.

The dose is ½ to 1 teaspoonful of the liquid extract of the bark in water three times daily.

A very useful prescription is as follows:-

  ½oz Prickly Ash bark
  ½oz Guaiacum raspings
  ½oz Buckbean herb
  6 Cayenne pods

Boil in 1½ pints of water down to 1 pint. A wineglassful may be taken three or four times daily.

In his book, The Natural Home Physician, Eric F.W. Powell recommends the following formula:-

Burdock herb	½oz
Prickly Ash berries	½oz
Guaiacum chips	½oz
Stinging nettles	½oz

This mixture should be simmered in two pints of water in an enamel or stainless steel saucepan for twenty minutes. When strained a large wineglassful should be taken before meals.

This prescription has proved very effective in many cases of rheumatism and fibrositis.

The Herbal Therapeutic Index on page 77 should be helpful.

HEALTH GIVING
HERBAL TEAS

The following herbs can be made into teas or tisanes and taken daily instead of the usual Indian tea.

They are delicious and health giving and were used extensively in olden days.

Any tea that helps to promote bowel action, aid digestion or purify the blood is in turn helping the body to overcome the pains of rheumatism.

If any sweetening is necessary a little honey may be added.

Many herbal tisanes are available packed in tea bags for easy handling, otherwise the tea should be made in the usual way. The pot should be warmed and boiling water poured onto the herb; two teaspoonsful to one pint of water. This should steep for five minutes before drinking.

Bergamot Tea
The Oswego Indians drank this tea and when the American colonists boycotted British tea they also drank Bergamot which they called Oswego tea.

This tea is soothing and relaxing and should be taken last thing at night as it promotes sleep.

This tea should be simmered for ten minutes to enhance the flavour. One teaspoonful of the herb per cup.

Chamomile Tea
This is a pleasing flavour and a tisane still drunk by many in France as it aids digestion and is very effective after a heavy meal. It is also a sedative and tonic and is helpful to ease neuralgic pains.

Dandelion Tea
This tea improves rheumatic conditions, as well as influencing the liver and gall bladder.

Lemon Balm Tea
This is a delicious tea and has many uses. Most important as far as the readers of this book are concerned is that it removes spasms and tension, and because of this sleep comes more easily.

It has the reputation of helping the memory and removing depression.

It is recommended first thing in the morning as it counteracts tiredness, helping the one who has taken it to rise feeling better than without it.

Lime Flower Tea (Tilleul)
This is another delicious tea which is very popular in France; it has a delicate flavour.

This tea soothes the nerves and allays spasms; it is also helpful in digestive troubles.

If taken last thing at night it will help to promote sleep because the nerves are calmed.

Mint Tea
All the mints make delicious teas, the most

popular being peppermint.

When tired this is useful as a pick-me-up and it is also recommended for cramps. It is mostly used for indigestion after a meal.

Parsley Tea
This is a delicious tea and most helpful if used daily as it contains vitamins A, B, and C.

It is a tonic herb and is valuable as a diuretic which helps to rid the body of too much fluid.

It has long been recommended for rheumatism.

Rose Hip Tea
This is excellent owing to its content of vitamin C.

Rose hip and Hibiscus tea is packed in tea bags commercially and is delicious. The hibiscus gives the tea a rich pink colour and exciting lemon flavour. It is very pleasant.

Sage Tea
Another delicious tea which has disinfectant properties. It is useful in rheumatism and helps to stimulate the circulation.

Chapter 8

EPSOM SALTS BATHS

Epsom Salts Baths are important and most beneficial and they should be taken regularly by all who suffer from rheumatism or arthritis.

Crude Epsom Salts can be purchased in 7lb bags relatively cheaply.

Between 1 and 2lbs of Epsom Salts should be dissolved in a bath half filled with hot water and the patient should soak in this for about ten minutes. The temperature of the water should be controlled to suit each patient. During this ten minutes the body should be constantly rubbed all over with a skin brush or loofah. This removes the waste matter which exudes through the skin and unless frequent rubbing is continued the pores of the skin become clogged with the first waste matter and no more can be drawn out.

After ten minutes the water and deposits should be emptied away and replaced with clean warm water with which the body should be rubbed down. A pure soap may be used if desired.

It is a good thing to have this bath and then get into bed, and if possible in between flannelette sheets; otherwise the patient should be rolled in a thin blanket.

Patients suffering from heart conditions or high blood pressure, etc., should not take a full Epsom Salts bath but they can make use of compresses.

A piece of pure linen (white) should be dipped into a bowl of cold water containing a handful of Epsom Salts. This should be wrung out and applied to the affected part and immediately covered snugly with a warm woollen scarf, and fastened in place. This should be left on all night. The action of the warm wool should heat up the area at once and this stimulates circulation through the joint, blood and lymph. If the area does not begin to feel warm soor after the woollen covering has been fixed, remove the linen at once and wash the surface in warm water, otherwise a chill will follow.

The linen should be washed, boiled and dried ready for the next compress.

If the trouble occurs in the elbows, arms, legs or knees, the compress would be beneficial applied to the affected part twice a week, in addition to the Epsom Salt bath.

Foot baths also, should be considered. The patient should sit with feet in a bowl of hot water to which has been added 4oz of Epsom Salts. The feet should be rubbed with a loofah or skin brush at intervals as poisons will be drawn out through the feet. A kettle of hot water should be at hand in order that the temperature of the water may be kept up. After about 15 minutes the feet should be washed in warm water and a little vegetable oil massaged into the skin. The patient should stay in a warm temperature or get into a warm bed after this foot bath as very often the body sweats from the heat of the water.

Chapter 9

AVOID CONSTIPATION

Many people suffer from constipation, and it is essential that those suffering from arthritis and rheumatism realize the importance of getting the bowels in good working order.

Waste products and toxic matter should be eliminated freely and the adjustment of the daily diet, as advised in chapter 4 often puts things right.

When constipation is of long standing, however, the bowel has to be re-educated.

It is helpful to take, first thing in the morning, the juice of half a lemon plus a tablesspoonful of cold water in which have been soaked overnight a dozen raisins. After drinking the liquid the raisins should be thoroughly chewed and eaten.

Breakfast is an important meal in the cure of constipation. Bulk is necessary if bowel activity is to be induced and this can come from a dessertspoonful or two of muesli (according to one's appetite) and one of wheat germ into which is grated pears or apples unpeeled. These should be compost grown if possible. Ripe berries may be added when in season. When no fresh fruit is available, sun-dried fruit soaked overnight may be added - apricots, pears, prunes or raisins.

A little honey is the very best natural sweetner and good for the heart; it also provides heat and energy.

Diluted fruit juice or a little plain yoghourt may be added to complete a nourishing and health-giving breakfast which should, in time, help the bowels to work freely. If only pasteurised milk is obtainable then a little plain yoghourt may be used instead. This is best obtained from a health food store and a reliable make purchased. The original and best yoghourt is obtained from goat's milk and this can often be found.

As a matter of interest constipating foods include white bread, pastries, cakes and biscuits made from white flour, spaghetti and macaroni, pasteurised milk, polished rice, tapioca and sago, custard made from powder, pickles, etc.

Foods which help to promote healthy bowel function are most root and all green, leafy vegetables, yoghourt, bran, crude black molasses, whole grain cereals, most ripe fruits in season, wheat germ and dried brewer's yeast.

All aperients should be stopped except one of the herbal preparations - never use liquid paraffin.

A small teaspoonful of sunflower seed or soya oil is helpful in some cases if oil can be tolerated, taken 3 times daily just before meals. This should **not** be taken last thing at night.

It is essential that the patient should go to stool at the same time each day. No straining should take place but this regular habit will prove beneficial after a time.

Overcoming constipation is a great step in the right direction and the sooner this is achieved the better.

Chapter 10

THE NEW ZEALAND GREEN-LIPPED MUSSEL

I feel it is important to say something about the Green-Lipped Mussel which is playing its part in helping some patients with arthritis to improve and live a fuller and less painful life.

All the known minerals are in the sea, just as they are in our bodies, and we do not have to stretch our imaginations too far to accept that quantities of these minerals become absorbed by all marine life.

Seaweeds have been used by natural healers with excellent results for many decades; indeed, I have written on the merits of Kelp in chapter eleven.

The Green-Lipped Mussel has its home in the comparatively unpolluted waters around the coasts of New Zealand and it is now cultivated in farms in order that supplies of top quality mussels are obtained. A substance is extracted from these shell fish at a specific time, and after complicated processes this is made up into capsules or tablets.

A great deal of research was done in the late 1960's and early 1970's when it was found that the mussel extract had an anti-arthritic action. The first experiments were carried out on rats.

Results of some clinical trials were published in 'The Practioner' which said that the extract 'is an effective supplement or possible alternative to orthodox therapy in the treatment of rheumatoid and osteo-arthritis.

Sixty-six patients took part in these trials, twenty eight suffering from rheumatoid arthritis and thirty eight from osteo-arthritis. 67.9% of these patients with rheumatoid arthritis and 39.5% of those with osteo-arthritis felt some benefit from the treatment. The improvements during the trial included less pain, less stiffness and the ability to cope.

Less pain and more mobility are the two symptoms reported by many patients and this improved state can last for some months when another course of treatment may be necessary. On the other hand the improvement may not deteriorate. No two patients are alike and therefore some may need more doses of the mussel extract than others. At the same time, some patients may react very much more quickly than others. And some will get no benefit at all.

At this point I must stress that this is not a cure for every arthritic sufferer.

There is a warning that people who are allergic to sea-foods should not take the Green-Lipped Mussel treatment - this is important.

There may be an aggravation of symptoms early in the course of treatment, but this usually means that an improvement will follow.

The Green-Lipped Mussel extract can be obtained from any Health Food Store.

Chapter 11

SUPPLEMENTARY ADVICE

Our Daily Bread

The writer has taught many people to make bread and they have been delighted with results, particularly as it is so quick and easy.

Most people groan at the idea of bread making, possibly because it conjures up memories of their mothers kneading the dough several times and the making of it seemed to take so long.

Always remember that the best bread is made in a warm kitchen with warm utensils. This is the recipe:

> 3 lbs stone-ground 100 per cent wholemeal flour
> 2 pints luke warm water
> 1 flat dessertspoonful sea salt
> 1 dessertspoonful barbados sugar
> 3 tablespoons sunflower or soya oil
> 1 oz fresh or desiccated yeast

Warm a large basin, tip in the flour, add the salt and mix well in a warm place.

Put the yeast into a small basin (crumble if fresh), add sugar and about a quarter of a pint of the warm water. Leave this in a warm place until it becomes frothy, which should take only a few minutes.

Then 3 two pint loaf tins should be well greased with dripping if possible as other fats are more liable to stick. Put tins in a warm place.

When the yeast is ready make a well in the flour, stir the yeast and sugar and pour on to flour. Add 3 tablespoonsful of oil and mix well with the hands. It should leave the side of the bowl clean but, at the same time, be moist.

Divide the dough into three, place in the tins and then put the 3 tins somewhere warm to enable the dough to rise. A shelf above a low gas flame is ideal, or in a plate warming drawer, or even in a warm airing cupboard. The tins should be covered. The dough should be left to rise to the top of the tin (about twenty minutes or so) and then baked for 35 to 45 minutes in an oven at 425F if electric and at Regulo No.6 if gas.

When cooked the loaf should sound hollow when rapped with the knuckles.

The bread should be left to settle for 24 hours before cutting. It will keep far longer than bought bread although the writer finds that home-made bread disappears far more quickly than any other.

For a change, add a few raisins and a little barbados sugar to one third of the dough — mix throughly and put into tin and leave to rise, then bake in the usual way. It may take a little longer to get to the top of the tin. This is a great favourite for afternoon tea!

Cod Liver Oil

Osteo arthritis is a joint disease and although books have been written on the subject, with many different opinions, most agree that there is wear in the joint when the synovial fluid decreases. Some patients have said that the joint feels rough and 'if only some oil could be injected I feel it would be eased'.

Many experts in nutrition say that if bones crumble or deposits of calcium are found, this means that calcium is not being assimilated, and in turn this may be a pointer that insufficient vitamin D is present. Cod liver oil is taken by patients suffering from osteo arthritis as it provides this vitamin which helps bone formation and this could improve the condition.

Another interesting factor here is that research shows that there is a connection between a high concentration of cholesterol in the blood and osteo arthritis. Cod liver oil is an unsaturated fat and would therefore be effective in lowering blood cholesterol levels.

We all know that cod liver oil capsules help to keep colds at bay if taken during the winter months, so it would seem to be a very useful additive to the daily diet.

Exercise

Walking is one of the best exercises because it can be regulated to suit the patient's capabilities. Obviously this is out of the question for many suffering from rheumatism or arthritis, but if possible a walk every day in the fresh air is recommended. The question is always asked, 'How far should I go?' and the simple answer must be, 'As far as you are able'. In other words it is wrong for anybody to make up his mind to walk a mile regardless of whether he is really fit enough to do so. A patient should walk (at his own pace) just as far as he feels able to do so comfortably without getting overtired, or pushing himself to do so. Deep breathing should be enjoyed at the same time and this will give great benefit.

If a patient cannot walk it may be possible to exercise the limb that is suffering; or in the case of stiff hands and fingers, moving them as though playing a piano, or squeezing a small ball, often keeps the hands mobile.

Naturally, it is necessary to use common sense about exercise especially where rheumatic and arthritic patients are concerned. Avoid walking in rain and getting wet. Strong winds can also be harmful. Try to take outdoor exercise during the warmest part of the day in winter and in summer avoid great heat.

Fresh Air

Breathing fresh air is most important although it does not appear to have a bearing on rheumatic ailments, but it should be borne in mind that in order to resist disease it is necessary to build up the general health, and fresh air plays an important part in this effort.

All rooms should be well ventilated, and bedrooms should have a window open at night except when there is fog about.

Deep breathing at an open window, according to one's physical ability is excellent as it enables the body to take in oxygen which, as everyone knows, is a vital factor in life itself. However, avoid draughts and hot, stuffy rooms which are harmful.

Juices

Carrot and celery juice are very good indeed for patients suffering from arthritis or rheumatism.

The juice of 3 ozs of raw carrot and 1 oz of celery should be extracted and taken before lunch or mid-morning. This help to counteract acidity.

In addition to the above the juice of spinach, parsley, lettuce, watercress and cucumber are recommended for rheumatism, and for arthritis beetroot and cucumber.

Kelp (Fucus vesiculosus)

This plant of the sea should be studied with care for it has helped many patients suffering from all kinds of troubles.

It contains iodine, calcium, phosphorus, iron, sodium, potassium, magnesium, sulphur, chlorine, copper, zinc and manganese. There are also traces of barium, boron, chromium, lithium, nickel, silver, titanium, vanadium, aluminium, strontium and silicon. In addition some vitamins are found as well.

Kelp is indeed a good natural source of minerals and vitamins so vital to the human economy.

Taken every day, it not only helps to control the rheumatic diseases, but assists greatly in rebuilding and maintaining healthy body cells.

Many patients suffering from rheumatism are constipated and Eric Powell in his book on Kelp says he has never found a case of constipation that did not respond to a breakfast of soaked prunes, a little bran and a good pinch of kelp; a tumbler of hot water in which a small teaspoonful of molasses is dissolved should be sipped at the same meal. This has been found to be very beneficial in many cases.

Two or three kelp tablets should be taken with three meals daily and continued for long periods as this is a food supplement and not a medicine.

If possible, tablets in the 1x or 2x potency should be obtained (from any homeopathic chemist) as they are more easily assimilated and more pleasant to take.

Oils for massage

Massage is often helpful and olive or sun-flowerseed oil can be applied to any part of the body. Stiff and painful joints, fingers, thumbs, elbows, knees and feet can all be treated with benefit. Before massage the part should be bathed in hot water to open the pores and then the massage with the oil carried out in a gentle manner, very little pressure being used.

To obtain satisfactory results this must be done regularly once or twice daily over a long period.

Peanut oil is said to be very helpful if gently rubbed into the painful parts several times a week. It is particularly effective after a bath.

The late Samuel Thompson recommended a compound tincture of 1 teaspoonful tincture of Capsicum (cayenne) added to 2ozs tincture of Myrrh. This makes a good liniment and should be rubbed into the painful area of the body regularly.

Potato (Solanum tuberosum)

The potato contains large quantites of potash salts which makes it a valuable food providing it is cooked properly. To retain the important minerals potatoes must be cooked in their jackets. Potatoes baked in this way are delicious but they can be steamed in their skins and if desired the paper thin skin removed when they are hot, it can then be stripped off very easily and the salts will not be lost.

Fernie says, 'The carriage of a small raw potato in a trousers pocket has been often found preventive of rheumatism in a person predisposed thereto, probably by reason of the sulphur and the narcotic principles contained in the peel. Ladies in former times had their dresses supplied with special bags or pockets in which to carry one or more small raw potatoes about their person for avoiding rheumatism'.

Compresses made from grated raw potatoes mixed with a little milk and applied to the painful part aid in the elimination of pain and inflammation.

If a cold compress is not desirable, potatoes boiled in their skins should be mashed up and whilst still hot mixed with a little milk and applied to the affected part in between two pieces of muslin. This is best done on going to bed when it can remain all night.

The juice of a small potato diluted is very beneficial to rheumatic conditions as it is highly alkaline and is therefore an effective antidote to uric acid.

If potato juice is not palatable it may be added to soups, but care should be taken not to cook the juice with the soup.

Chapter 12

THE IMPORTANCE OF
THINKING POSITIVELY

Positive or creative thought is the most powerful and important factor in our lives.

Most people take 'thinking' for granted — thoughts are just thoughts, they come and they go — so what are we bothered about?

We are referring to MIND USE which is such a dominant factor in health and healing.

"We are what we think" is a very old and true axiom. Many years ago Dr. Coue healed countless people of many diseases by teaching them to think positively and repeating twenty times each day 'Every day and in every way I feel better and better'. Coue's repeated sentence meant that the mind was controlled, thought was positive and the result — healing was taking place in the physical body reaching every tiny cell.

The power of thought is mind boggling. Positive thought heals and conversely negative thinking fills our bodies with poisons and disease develops. Our thoughts are reflected in our bodies all of the time.

This I realise is a new concept for some people and difficult to accept. But there are one or two illustrations which may be helpful. For instance, if we suffer a great shock we often say 'It went straight to my stomach and I felt sick'. The shock was absorbed by the mind and this produced discomfort in the stomach and the feeling of sickness. And if somebody says 'You do look weary and tired today' then the person concerned **feels** tired and disheartened because these negative thoughts have affected her. On the other hand if somebody who is not well meets a friend who says 'How lovely to see you and you're looking so much better' that happy, creative thought is healing and enters into the one who is unwell and she feels so much better.

From these examples we can understand that we all affect each other. Sometimes without even saying anything we can feel happy and comfortable with somebody and very different with another person. And this brings me to a very important point. We should all remember that all our thoughts are very powerful, they not only affect us but those around us.

Many of you reading this will be suffering pain; it is understandable that you become depressed and perhaps a bit irritable and even feel that life is not worth living. But this is an attitude of defeat and the very depression and perhaps resentment, cause more poisons to be released into the bloodstream, thus adding fuel to the fires of disease. I have every sympathy for people who are suffering and I know that constant pain is very wearing. This is why I want to help.

Changing our thoughts from negative to positive is not easy but it can be managed with practise and resolution. The first thing is to focus your thoughts on something outside of yourself — recognise a sunny day and say 'how lovely everything looks in the sunshine, I'm going to enjoy today'. Immediately your pain will not be quite so bad and **you** will feel happier. Or think of all the things for which you are grateful (we all have some if we look for them) and say 'thank you'. This is another positive statement!

There is much that you can do for yourself. At the beginning of each day if you sit quietly and think of 'PEACE' – that you are full of peace; that you are in a peaceful place – perhaps you can visualize walking along by the sea as the waves lap gently on the sand, or on soft grass by a river where the wild flowers grow and birds sing overhead; you will begin to feel an inner peace and healing will be taking place.

All this and much more is taught and discussed in 'The ABC of Health & Healing' by Jack Burton, M.A., and can be obtained from Book Dept., Maillard House Trust, Manor House, Coffinswell, Newton Abbot, Devon, TQ12 4SW price £6.00 including postage.

This is a book to be read and re-read because it teaches us to heal ourselves and other people. Jack has been healing the sick for thirty years and he shares his knowledge and experiences.

Today we are learning more and more about the power of the mind and I am introducing it to you because it has helped so many people who are sick and I hope that you too will benefit.

Do not give up. You can do so much to help yourself and creative thought is the most important of all the 'Do's' that I have mentioned in these pages.

ABBREVIATIONS

Actea spicata. **Ac.spic.**
Ammonium Carbonicum. **Amm.c.**
Antimonium tartaricum. **Ant.t.**
Arnica montana. **Arn.**
Arsenicum album. **Ars.alb.**
Bryonia album. **Bry.**
Calcarea carbonica. **Calc.c.**
Caulophyllum. **Caul.**
Causticum. **Caust.**
Cimicifuga. **Cim.**
Colchicum. **Colch.**
Colocynthis. **Coloc.**
Eupatorium perfoliatum. **Eup.perf.**
Gelsemium. **Gels.**
Gnaphalium. **Gnaph.**
Hepar sulphuris. **Hep.sulph.**
Ledum palustre. **Led.**
Magnesia Carbonica. **Mag.c.**
Natrum muriaticum. **Nat.m.**
Nux vomica. **Nux.v.**
Phytolacca. **Phyt.**
Pulsatilla. **Puls.**
Ranunculus bulb. **Ran.b.**
Rhododendron. **Rhod.**
Rhus toxicodendron. **Rhus.t.**
Ruta graveolens. **Ruta.**
Sanguinaria canadensis. **Sang.**
Sulphur. **Sulph.**

HERBAL THERAPEUTIC INDEX

ARTHRITIS: Dandelion, Nettle
ARTHRITIS, RHEUMATOID: Guaiacum
BLOOD PURIFIER: Burdock, Celery, Centaury, Dandelion, Guaiacum, Nettle, Prickly Ash
GOUT: Birch, Goutweed, Guaiacum, Horseradish compress
INFLAMMATIONS, TO SOOTHE: Hops fomentation
JOINTS, PAINFUL: Goutweed
LAXATIVE: Dandelion
PAINS, MUSCULAR: Hops fomentation
PAINS, RHEUMATIC: Goutweed compress
RHEUMATISM: Birch, Burdock, Celery, Dandelion, Goutweed
RHEUMATISM, CHRONIC: Guaiacum, Horseradish compress, Prickly Ash
RHEUMATISM, MUSCULAR: Centaury, Hops fomentation
SCIATICA: Horseradish compress
SWELLINGS, PAINFUL: Juniper berries
URIC ACID, REMOVES: Dandelion, Juniper berries
URIC ACID, SOLVENT: Nettle

GLOSSARY OF
MEDICAL TERMS

ANODYNE. Pain easing.

APERIENT. Producing a natural movement of the bowels.

AROMATIC. Having an aroma.

ASTRINGENT. Binding. Causing contraction of the tissues.

BITTER. Applied to bitter-tasting drugs which are used to stimulate the appetite.

CARMINATIVE. Easing griping pains and expelling flatulence.

DIAPHORETIC. Drugs which promote perspiration.

DIURETIC. Eliminates water from the system.

SEDATIVE. Drugs which calm nervous excitement.

STOMACHIC. Applied to drugs given for disorders of the stomach.

TONIC. Substances which give tone to the body producing a feeling of well-being.

FOR FURTHER READING

HOMOEOPATHY FOR EMERGENCIES by Phyllis Speight, pub by Health Science Press

HOMOEOPATHY FOR THE FIRST-AIDER by Dr. D. Shepherd, pub by Health Science Press

HOMOEOPATHY, A PRACTICAL GUIDE TO NATURAL MEDICINE by Phyllis Speight, pub by Granada Publishing Co Ltd

NEW HOPE FOR ARTHRITICS by Dong & Banks, pub by Granada Publishing Co Ltd

RELIEF FROM ARTHRITIS – THE STORY OF THE GREEN-LIPPED MUSSEL by J.E. Croft, pub by Thorsons Publishers Ltd

TAKING THE ROUGH WITH THE SMOOTH by Dr. A. Stanway, pub by Pan Books

THE A.B.C. OF HEALTH & HEALING by Jack Burton, pub by Maillard House Trust, Manor House, Coffinswell, Newton Abbot, Devon

THE ARTHRITICS COOK BOOK by Dong & Banks, pub by Granada Publishing Co Ltd

HOMOEOPATHIC INDEX OF SYMPTOMS

CAUSE

Exposure to cold, dry winds. **Hep. sulph.**

Exposure to stormy weather. **Rhod.**

Exposure to damp and cold. **Arn.**

Getting wet. **Puls.**

Getting feet wet. **Puls.**

Injury to bones. **Ruta.**

News, bad. **Gels.**

Over-exertion. **Arn.**

Over-lifting. **Calc.c.**

Over-straining. **Calc.c., Rhus.t.**

Working in water. **Calc.c.**

CONCOMITANT

Better by heat. **Rhus.t.**

Better by holding feet in ice cold water. **Led.**

Better by motion. **Coloc., Gels.**

Better by rubbing. **Rhus.t.**

Better from warm, moist air. **Caust.**

Better warmed by exercise. **Rhus.t.**

Better by warmth. **Amm.c., Hep. sulph., Mag.c.**

Worse ascending. **Calc.c.**

Worse change of temperature. **Mag.c.**

Worse change of weather. **Calc.c., Ran.b.**

Worse cold. **Caust. Nux.v.**

Worse cold applications. **Ruta.**

Worse cold, damp weather. **Colch., Rhod., Ruta.**

Worse cold, wet weather. **Calc.c., Rhus.t.**

Worse cold, dry air. **Hep. sulph.**

Worse cold winds. **Hep.sulph.**

Worse cold, dry winds. **Caust.**

Worse damp weather. **Phyt., Rhus.t.**

Worse draughts. **Mag.c., Rhus.t.**

Worse eating, after. **Calc.c.**

Worse evening. **Bry., Caust., Led., Ran.b.**

Worse heat and cold. **Colch.**

Worse hot weather. **Puls., Sang., Sulph.**

Worse lifting. **Sang.**

Worse lying on painful side. **Bry.**

Worse morning. **Bry., Calc.c., Eup. perf.**

Worse motion. **Ac.spic., Arn., Bry., Calc.c., Cim., Coloc., Led., Phyt., Rhod., Sang.**

Worse night. **Ac.spic., Hep.sulph., Nat.m., Phyt., Puls., Sang., Sulph.**

Worse sitting. **Nat.m., Phyt., Rhus.t., Ruta.**

Worse stormy weather. **Ran.b., Rhod.**

Worse thunderstorms. **Rhod.**

Worse touch. **Ac.spic., Colch.**

Worse turning in bed. **Nux.v., Sang.**

Worse vexation. **Rhod.**

Worse warmth. **Amm.c., Hep.sulph., Mag.c., Puls.**

Worse walking. **Nat.m.**

Worse wet weather. **Amm.c.**

Worse when beginning to move. **Rhus.t.**

Worse wind. **Rhod.**

PAINS

in ankles. **Ac.spic., Caul., Nat.m., Ruta.**

in arms. **Bry., Caust., Cim., Colch., Coloc., Eup.perf., Hep.sulph., Phyt., Puls., Rhod., Sang.**

in back. **Amm.c., Ant.t., Ars.alb., Calc.c., Caust., Cim., Eup.perf., Gels.,**

Gnaph., Hep.sulph., Nat.m., Nux.v.,
Phyt., Puls., Ran.b., Rhod., Rhus.t.,
Ruta., Sang., Sulph.

in calves. Ant.t., Calc.c.

in elbows. Ac.spic., Eup.perf., Rhus.t.

in extremities. Ant.t., Coloc.

in feet. Arn., Caust., Colch., Coloc.,
Mag.c., Puls., Rhus.t.

in finger joints. Ac.spic., Caul., Caust.,
Nat.m., Rhus.t.

in hands. Ac.spic., Caust., Colch.,
Coloc., Rhus.t.

in head. Eup.perf.

in heels. Amm.c., Bry.

in hips. Ant.t., Bry., Caust., Coloc.,
Nat.m., Puls., Rhod., Rhus.t., Ruta.

in intercostal muscles. Bry., Ran.b.

in joints (large). Nux.v.

in knees. Amm.c., Calc.c., Caust.,
Coloc., Eup.perf., Hep.sulph., Mag.
c., Nat.m., Phyt., Puls.

in legs. Arn., Caust., Gels., Mag.c.

in leg, bones of. Phyt.

in limbs, all. Caust., Rhod.

in muscles, abdominal. Ran.b.

in neck. Ars.alb., Amm.c., Cim.,
Colch., Eup.perf., Gels., Nat.m.,
Phyt., Puls., Sang.

in shoulder. Ars.alb., Bry., Calc.c.,
Caust., Colch., Coloc., Gels., Hep.
sulph., Mag.c., Nat.m., Nux.v., Phyt.,
Puls., Ran.b., Rhod., Rhus.t., Sang.,
Sulph.

in thighs. Ant.t., Caust., Coloc., Hep.
sulph., Nat.m.

in thumbs. Coloc.

in toes. Ac.spic., Caul., Led.

in toe, ball of big. Amm.c., Colch.,
Eup.perf., Nat.m.

Under toe-nails. Eup.perf.

in wrists. **Ac.spic., Calc.c., Caul., Eup.perf., Rhod., Rhus.t., Ruta.**
moving from joint to joint. **Colch.**
moving one place to another. **Caul., Puls.**
in sciatic nerve. **Gnaph.**
Better by perspiration. **Eup.perf.**

RESTLESSNESS
of limbs. **Ars.alb., Rhus.t.**
at night. **Caust.**

STIFFNESS
of ankles. **Sulph.**
of arthritic joints. **Bry.**
of back. **Caust., Phyt., Rhus.t.**
of feet. **Ars.alb., Rhus.t.**
of fingers. **Hep.sulph.**
of joints. **Ac.spic., Cim., Coloc.**
of knees. **Ars.alb., Rhus.t.**
of limbs. **Nat.m.**
of lower limbs. **Eup.perf**
of neck. **Ars.alb., Calc.c., Caust., Cim., Colch., Coloc., Nux.v., Phyt., Rhod., Rhus.t.**
of shoulders. **Rhus.t.**

SWELLING
of ankles. **Caul., Hep.sulph.**
of arms. **Bry.**
of feet. **Arn., Bry., Led., Puls.**
of fingers. **Caul., Hep.sulph., Mag.c., Rhus.t.**
of hands. **Amm.c., Calc.c., Hep.sulph., Puls., Rhus.t.**
of heels. **Bry.**
of joints. **Calc.c., Led.**
of joints, arthritic. **Bry., Sang.**
of joints of big toe. **Arn.**
of joints, small. **Ac.spic.**

of knee. **Amm.c., Calc.c., Led., Mag. c., Puls., Sulph.**
of knee joint. **Bry., Hep.sulph.**
of legs. **Arn., Led.**
of muscles. **Bry.**
of neck. **Nat.m.**
of shoulders. **Bry.**
of toes. **Amm.c., Caul.**
of toes, ball of big. **Led.**
of toe, big. **Amm.c.**
of wrists. **Caul.**

WEAKNESS
of back. **Eup.perf.**
of limbs. **Caust.**
of lower limbs. **Amm.c.**

INDEX